Postural Tachycardia Syndrome

(POTS)

All That You Need to Know

Fhilcar Faunillan

Table of Contents

INTRODUCTION i

CHAPTER 1: 1

Understanding Postural 1

Tachycardia Syndrome 1

   The Prevalence of POTS 7

CHAPTER 2: 10

Triggers and Symptoms of POTS...............................10

   Symptoms of POTS 12

   Triggers of POTS...17

CHAPTER 3: 30

Causes and Types of POTS...30

   Causes of POTS 30

   Health Conditions That May Lead to POTS..............34

   Types of POTS 36

      Primary POTS 37

      Secondary POTS 39

      Hypovolemic and Neuropathic POTS 42

CHAPTER 4: 44

Diagnosing Postural 44

Tachycardia Syndrome 44

   Criteria for an Accurate Diagnosis of POTS 47

Active Stand or Poor Man's Tilt................................ 48

Tilt Table 48

24-Hour BP and Heart Rate Monitoring 49

Isoproterenol Administration................................. 50

24-Hour Urine Test 51

Blood Tests... 51

Heart Ultrasound (Echocardiogram) 52

Microneurography... 52

Holter Monitor 53

Hand Grip Test.. 54

Sweat Tests 54

Stress Test 56

Catecholamine Test 57

Chapter 5: 59

Lifestyle Adjustments and Medications for POTS 59

Lifestyle Adjustments 60

Drink More Fluids Regularly 61

Maintain Good Body Posture 62

Increase Salt Intake.. 63

Eat the Right Foods 64

Regulate Temperatures 64

Wear Compression Clothing................................ 65

Elevate Your Head during Sleep 65

Match Physical Activities with Your Capabilities .. 66

Manage Personal Hygiene 68

Plan in Advance...68

Adopt Good Work and Reading Habits 69

Use a Mobility Scooter or Wheelchair 69

Keep Your Tools in One Place 70

List Your Medication and Create Reminders 71

Medications for POTS...72

Drugs to Regulate Heart Rate 73

Medications to Boost Blood Volume....................76

CHAPTER 6: 78

POTS Prognosis 78

Conclusion 80

INTRODUCTION

The main purpose of this book is to provide you with useful information about Postural Tachycardia Syndrome (POTS). The medicine industry has undergone significant changes in recent years due to the efforts of health practitioners and the inception of new technology. In the past, it was difficult to cure some cancer conditions, but things have changed over the years. It is now possible to treat some of these conditions if diagnosed in their initial stages of development. Persons with disabilities are now able to move thanks to advanced prosthetics. The bottom line is that many patients can now smile because they can be saved from life-threatening health problems and complications.

Advanced medical studies have helped researchers discover treatments for a wide range of health problems including severe health conditions. However, some health problems still affect millions of patients across the globe even after many years of research. Postural Tachycardia Syndrome is one of those health problems. Even though POTS is not a life-threatening syndrome, it can affect your quality of life by limiting your capability to engage in everyday physical activities. Another problem with POTS is that the chances of misdiagnosing the condition are high and getting the right treatment can be troublesome.

Luckily, after the many years of researching, observing, and assessing patients with POTS, a lot of information has been gathered to help patients live a better life. If you have the syndrome or know someone who has it, then you are reading the right book. In this book, you will learn more about POTS. As you read through each section of the book, you will learn the ABC's of POTS and find out more about how to manage the syndrome.

You will also learn about the history of POTS and the methods medical doctors have been using to deal with the syndrome. This book explains what POTS is in simple terms and helps the reader know the people who are most likely to have the condition. You need this information so you can be aware and help patients including your loved ones. Read on to learn more about the causes of POTS, the different types of POTS, and some common health problems related to the syndrome. Additionally, you will find out how POTS may affect the patients suffering from this condition depending on their age.

As mentioned earlier, health practitioners often misdiagnose POTS and the best way to avoid this problem is to know the symptoms. This book will explain the symptoms experienced by those suffering from the syndrome. You will learn how individual patients may experience varied symptoms depending on various factors including their age group. Also, you will discover the potential triggers of the syndrome and learn about some simple solutions to help patients alleviate the symptoms.

Those afflicted with POTS must fulfill certain criteria for an accurate diagnosis of the syndrome to be performed. This book will discuss the criteria you need to meet for a physician to confirm that you have POTS. You will also find useful information about the tests your physician needs to perform to confirm the diagnosis. These include tests like the Catecholamine test and the Tilt Table Test.

If you undergo the appropriate diagnostic procedures and there is no doubt that you have POTS, your life may take a different turn and you have to take the necessary measures. In this book, we will talk about the measures you need to take if you are suffering from POTS. Hopefully, the adjustments recommended here will help you become functional as before or help to improve the lives of others who could be having the syndrome including the people you love.

This book also focuses on the different types of medications for patients with POTS. Moreover, you will learn about the side effects of POTS medications and the steps you can take to prevent or reduce them. This information is important because those suffering from POTS experience the symptoms and side effects differently.

Overall, this book is for you if you have POTS and for any person who wants to help patients diagnosed with the syndrome. It will help you if you are looking after a POTS patient. Read it to learn everything you need to know about POTS and use the information provided here to help those afflicted with the syndrome. POTS patients have difficult moments living with the syndrome and you can help them if you have the appropriate knowledge. This book will prepare you to be ready all the time so you can help POTS patients who might need your help.

CHAPTER 1:

Understanding Postural Tachycardia Syndrome

Some of the things we do every day like standing, breathing, and blinking may look simple and it is easy for many people to take them for granted. Standing is one of the simplest daily routines which have been around for many years. However, it is not as simple as it looks because it involves the functions of various, complex systems that enable us to stand effortlessly. When you are standing, sitting or lying down, your body has to keep everything balanced and react to the earth's gravitational pull.

However, we usually don't think about the complex combinations of body systems and that is why we take standing for granted. The seemingly simple act of standing can be extremely difficult for some people due to various reasons. For instance, some people have difficulty standing because of health disorders that interfere with the body's ability to react to the earth's gravitational force when they try to change positions. Postural Tachycardia Syndrome is one of such disorders.

Let us look at two examples to help you understand what it means to have the syndrome. In the first scenario, you are waking up in the morning as usual only to realize that you are twenty minutes late. You want to get ready for work or school as quickly as possible, so you stand up swiftly (from supine position to upright position). A few seconds later, you start feeling dizzy and your heart rate is higher than normal. In an attempt to recover your composure, you decide to take some deep breaths.

Studies have revealed that this feeling is normal. It occurs when your blood drops to your hands, feet, and belly due to the earth's gravitational pull. When this happens, your blood vessels become narrow and your heart beats faster than usual to make sure that blood flows to the heart and brain. This also reduces the risk of low blood pressure.

In the second scenario, you experience the same feeling when you get up from your bed in the morning, but it's more intense this time. You try to put your body in order only to start sweating or feel like fainting. If you notice these symptoms, you could be one of the millions of individuals who experience the symptoms of POTS across the globe.

So, what is Postural Tachycardia Syndrome? POTS refers to a circulatory disorder characterized by an abnormal increase in heart rate (tachycardia) when you change from a supine position to an upright position. It can occur after standing or sitting up. The unusual increase in heart rate emanates from the patient's autonomic nervous system (ANS), which regulates several bodily functions, responses, and organ systems. When you notice these changes, it means that your cardiovascular system is trying to keep blood flowing to your brain and maintain the normal blood pressure.

The abnormal increase in your heart rate means that your body is not able to maintain the correct blood pressure. This may occur if your blood vessel become tight or loose, or because of the degree of constriction experienced by a blood vessel (vascular tone or vascular resistance). The three factors responsible for maintaining normal blood pressure are heart rate, the heart's contraction force, and vascular resistance. Persons with POTS have vascular resistance problems.

Those suffering from the syndrome have blood vessels that are unable to maintain the normal degree of tightness. Moreover, their blood drops to the lower parts of the body, which makes the heart beat faster than usual and causes myocardial contractility. These compensations may help to maintain normal blood pressure, but they may not be enough for those suffering from POTS. They can lead to other symptoms including fatigue, difficulty breathing, and light-headedness. In serious cases, the patient might become unconscious. People with these symptoms often have an abnormal heart rate of more than 120 bpm or 40 bpm for persons aged between 12 and 19 when standing. The heart rate of a POTS patient may also increase by 30 beats per minute after 10 minutes from the normal heart rate.

Looking at the history of medicine and health problems, it is easy to notice that humans have been aware of Postural Tachycardia Syndrome for a long time. Additionally, people have used a wide range of names when referring to POTS. The most popular clinical names of the syndrome include Orthostatic Tachycardia, Mitral Valve Prolapse Syndrome, Chronic Orthostatic Intolerance, Soldier's Heart,

Neurocirculatory Asthenia, and DaCosta's Syndrome. The term POTS (meaning Postural Tachycardia Syndrome) was coined in 1993 by a Mayo Clinic neurologist called Dr. Philip Low.

The key defining feature of POTS is orthostatic intolerance, a condition characterized by symptoms that occur when standing upright and reduce when reclining. In patients with orthostatic intolerance, an excessively low amount of blood flows to the heart upon standing upright from a supine position. POTS patients are actually persons with Dysautonomia, a general term used when referring to disorders of the autonomic nerves system including POTS.

In addition to having an increased heart rate of more than 100 beats per minute (tachycardia), persons with POTS may experience other symptoms including chest pains, a feeling of dizziness, fainting, and purple hands or feet. Other symptoms of the condition include sweating, palpitations, and nausea. We will learn more about these symptoms in the following chapters of the book. A decrease in the normal blood pressure is a common symptom of POTS, but it is important to keep in mind that some patients may not show any changes in blood pressure. Also, the patient's blood pressure may increase or decrease depending on various factors. Due to the large number of symptoms that need to be considered, researchers concluded that medications that impair autonomic function should be excluded.

The Prevalence of POTS

Generally, the prevalence of POTS is unknown. However, it is estimated that up to three million Americans have been affected by the syndrome. It is also believed that millions of people in different parts of the world suffer from POTS. With the increasing number of POTS patients around the world, most technological developments and medical studies have focused on the causes and symptoms.

Studies have shown that people aged between 15 and 50 years can be affected by the syndrome regardless of their race or gender. However, some studies indicate that young women are at a higher risk of experiencing the symptoms of POTS than the rest of the population. According to recent studies, women are 5 times more likely to develop POTS compared to men. Although the condition affects both males and females, about 80% of all persons diagnosed with the syndrome are women. The condition can strike without a warning or develop gradually.

In some cases, the symptoms of POTS may improve or disappear within a short time. However, some patients have to deal with the symptoms for a long time. In the latter case, those affected by the syndrome can take various steps to reduce the occurrences and risks. The recommended strategy is to start with lifestyle changes before using any form of medicine.

There are many promising breakthroughs in the world of medicine giving researchers the motivation they need to do more research on the possible causes and treatments for POTS and other health problems. Today, most patients can learn about the condition and adapt before they undergo diagnostic procedures. After more than 20 years of research and hard work, we can now find useful information about an imbalanced ANS.

CHAPTER 2:

Triggers and Symptoms of POTS

The best way for health practitioners to accurately diagnose a health condition or illness is to evaluate the symptoms experienced by the patient. We have already mentioned that POTS affects millions of individuals in different parts of the world. Sadly, this number continues to increase every year and something must be done to help those affected by the syndrome. Whether you or someone else is the patient, it is crucial to detect the syndrome as early as possible and perform an accurate diagnosis.

The first step of an effective treatment process for POTS patients is to know the different types of symptoms experienced by those afflicted with the condition. As indicated earlier in this book, each patient experiences the symptoms of POTS differently. The symptoms can have serious, irregular, mild, or incremental effects. It is important to address them before they worsen. This chapter of the book will discuss the different symptoms you should watch out for to determine if you have POTS.

The symptoms experienced by one POTS patient may not be the same as those experienced by a different patient with the syndrome. This is because every person is unique and the effects of the syndrome affect each patient differently. Some patients only experience mild symptoms of POTS and can still go to school, work, and take part in physical, recreational, and social activities. Other patients have serious symptoms of POTS, which make it difficult to perform simple, everyday activities. If you are suffering from POTS you may have trouble standing still and it can be hard to stand upright without getting tired. You may also feel uncomfortable when you try to sit upright, eat something, do house chores, or accomplish personal tasks like bathing.

Symptoms of POTS

As discussed in the previous chapter, POTS is characterized by an abnormally high heart rate, especially when you try to stand from a spine to an upright position. Although this is the most common symptom of the syndrome, patients may also experience other symptoms.

Here is a list of some of the symptoms you are likely to experience if you have POTS:

- **Feeling Dizzy or Lightheaded** – If you have POTS, you will feel dizzy or lightheaded when you stand up from a sitting or supine position. You may also experience this symptoms if you sit for a long period.

- **Headaches** – An upright posture can contribute to low amounts of blood in the brain, which can in turn cause headaches. Research shows that 2 in every 3 POTS patients experience headaches.

- **Rapid, Strong, and Irregular Heartbeats** – These are commonly known as **palpitations** and may not be life-threatening. If you have palpitations, you will experience strong and rapid poundings in your chest.

- **Pain in the Chest** – It is not clear what the cause of chest pain is, but many POTS patients experience it. This type of pain is usually benign, but some people may experience severe pain in the chest when they try to stand upright.

- **Brain Fog** – Persons with this symptoms are unable to concentrate or think properly.

- **Breathing Problems** – One of the common symptoms of POTS is the inability to breathe properly or shortness of breath. This symptom is easy to notice when the patient tries to perform tasks that need a lot of effort. If the condition is severe, you may experience breathing problems when standing without doing anything.

- **Passing Out, Fainting or Syncope** – Fainting or syncope is a temporary loss of consciousness. Research shows that about 30% of patients diagnosed with POTS experience this symptom.

- **Exhaustion and Weakness** – POTS patients may feel exhausted and weak even without taking part in any form of physical activity. This is a common symptom of the syndrome and many patients say it can last for a long time.

- **Tremor or Shaking** – It is said that this symptom worsens when you are in an upright position. Some patients also claim to have cold feet and hands. Other patients claim to shake internally.

- **Lack of Sleep** – Many POTS patients have trouble falling asleep and often wake up with a rapidly beating heart. They usually wake up during the night and fall asleep again. Those suffering from POTS may also stay awake even if they sleep with their eyes closed. Various studies have established that poor sleep has a significant effect on an individual's mental health, physical health, and life in general.

- **Poor Vision** – Person with POTS may complain of visual problems including blurry or graying vision and vision with strong glares.

- **Anxiety** – Most POTS patients claim to experience panic attacks that need a diagnosis. However, anxiety and rapid or deep breathing (hyperventilation) often happens because of other symptoms of POTS and the fear of having the syndrome. Hyperventilation and anxiety may also occur if the patient is skeptical about the diagnosis.

- **Gut Problems** – The main symptoms of gut problems in POTS patient include bloating, early satiation, appetite loss, pain in the abdomen, nausea, diarrhea, and constipation.

Triggers of POTS

Today, we can answer many questions about POTS because of healthcare practitioners who have worked diligently to gather information about the syndrome. Medical advancements have also played an important role in answering some pressing questions about POTS. As mentioned earlier, people need to be aware of the triggers and the first symptoms of the syndrome to avoid complications. Now that we know some of the common symptoms of POTS, it is also important to know the possible triggers of the condition. Many medical studies have revealed that certain factors can worsen the situation, and these factors are what we call triggers. It is easy to manage and cure POTS if you are aware of the possible triggers of syndrome.

Here are some common triggers and the recommended solutions:

- **Alcohol** – Patients with POTS should stay away from drinks that contain alcohol. This is because alcohol content can dilate blood vessels leading to excessive body heat and sweating. Alcohol is also known to promote venous amalgamation and can cause intensified hypotension. Another problem with alcohol consumption is that it can cause dehydration.

- **Bending the Body** – In some cases, POTS symptoms occur when you try to pick up something on the ground from a siting or upright position. Instead of bending your waist to pick up something, try to kneel or squat.

- **Climbing Staircases** – You need a significant amount of effort to climb upstairs and this can worsen your situation if you have POTS. Instead of climbing staircases on your feet, take the escalator or elevator if possible.

- **Loss of Body Fluids (Dehydration)** — If you are suffering from POTS, you don't want to lose body fluids because the effects can be devastating. The chances of experiencing dizziness and headaches are high when you are dehydrated. For this reason, those suffering from POTS must always be hydrated.

- **Energy Drinks** — Persons with POSTS should avoid energy drinks. One volleyball player with POTS experienced a vasovagal reaction after drinking a popular energy drink. This example shows why you should stay away from such drinks.

- **Eating Large Meals** — When you eat large meals, a lot of blood can flow to your abdomen and exacerbate hypotension if you have been diagnosed with POTS.

- **Adrenaline (Epinephrine)** — Adrenaline can be used to treat a wide range of health conditions including cardiac arrest and superficial bleeding. It can also be used as numbing medication. The problem with adrenaline when it comes to POTS patients is that it can stimulate the heart, so those suffering from the syndrome should not use it.

- **Strenuous Physical Activity** – The truth is that some exercises can help POTS patients by preventing blood pooling in the abdomen. Exercises can also strengthen the patient's muscles. However, POTS patients are advised to consult with their doctors before engaging in physical exercises. If you have POTS, ask your physician to assess your physical fitness level to avoid exposing your body to a lot of pressure. POTS patients can aggravate the situation if they engage in strenuous exercises, so it is advisable to avoid such exercises.

- **Blood Donation** – It is perfectly fine to donate blood, but those suffering from POTS may endanger they life if they donate blood. Some of the patients diagnosed with POTS are hypovolemic or have reduced blood volume. Such patients need more blood and should not donate blood unless there is a serious medical cause. Also, blood donation can cause blood pooling in the patient's legs and lead to a low amount of blood in the brain and heart.

- **Lifting Heavy Objects** – If you often lift heavy objects, then you risk worsening the symptoms of POTS. When lifting a heavy object, the heart has to work harder than usual and this can lead to blood pooling in your lower limbs. This means that only a small amount of blood reaches your upper body muscles. According to one theory, pressure changes in some patients' cerebrospinal fluid can trigger the symptoms of POTS when lifting heavy objects.

- **High Temperatures** – High temperate is one of the common triggers of POTS. The problem with heat is that it can worsen the condition by dilating blood vessels and increasing peripheral venous pooling. With that in mind, POTS patients should not bask in the noon sun. Those suffering from the syndrome should also avoid hot tubs, greenhouses, spas, and saunas.

- **Eating Certain Types of Food** – Different types of food may trigger the symptoms of POTS. These include refined carbohydrates like sugar and white flour. These food can aggravate hypotension by increasing gut dilation. Some POTS patients also claim that certain dairy products have worsened their symptoms. The best way to know the appropriate food for you is to consult a dietician.

- **Flying on Airplanes** – Patients with POTS should be aware that the air we breathe during flights is usually dry. This means that those traveling on airplanes may feel dehydrated, and we have already learned that patients with POTS should avoid dehydration. If you have POTS, make sure you rehydrate your body before your airplane flights. In some rare occasions, POTS patients may experience blood pooling and develop blood clots in their legs. If you notice these symptoms every time you are on an airplane, ask the attendants for a bulkhead seat. This will allow you to keep your legs elevated and prevent the development of blood clots during your flight. You may also benefit from tights or compensation stockings. Hyperventilating could also be the cause of your problems while flying. If you didn't know, airplane cabins are usually pressurized to about 6,500 feet and this can lead to hyperventilation, especially if you have Dysautonomia. This means that you might experience more symptoms of POTS during your flight.

- **Too Much Stimulation** – The patient's environment can also aggravate the symptoms of POTS. For example, some patients claim that they are sensitive to loud noises, bright lights, and busy environments. These factors can worsen their problem and that is why some POTS patients choose to stay away from extremely stimulating environments.

- **Stress** – Another trigger that POTS patients should avoid is stress. If you are suffering from POTS, just do not force yourself to do the things you cannot do. Carry out your everyday activities to the best of your ability and avoid stressful activities that might aggravate the symptoms. Your body is naturally able to deal with mental, physical or chemical stress, but some POTS patients may not have this ability. This could be as a result of a malfunctioning or an excessively functioning ANS. Some POTS patients may also have high levels of norepinephrine, which is a stress hormone.

- **Lifting Hands Up** – If you have POTS and raise your hands up, you might trigger some of the symptoms of the syndrome. However, this only happens in some patients. When you lift up your arm, you heart may have difficulty pumping blood to every part of the raised arm and this can lead to tachycardia. Also, your heart has to pump harder than usual because of the increased gravitational pull when you hold your arms up. This can be a challenge if blood has already pooled in your lower limb veins.

- **Anesthesia** – In medicine, anesthesia is a state of temporary loss of sensation induced by health practitioners for medical purposes. However, this state can have negative effects on the body of a POTS patient, especially persons with autonomic dysfunction. This is because anesthesia can interfere with cardiovascular function.

- **Over-the-Counter Products** – Persons diagnosed with POTS may exacerbate their symptoms if they use products that claim to stimulate the heart or reduce blood pressure. For instance, caffeine is known to raise blood pressure when consumed by healthy people. However, caffeine can have devastating effects on the health status of a POTS patient in a hyperadrenergic state. It can be harmful when consumed by patients with high levels of excitation or anxiety. Also, those experiencing mixed feelings of nausea, nervousness, appetite loss, and shakiness may aggravate their symptoms if they consume products with caffeine. Moreover, caffeine is known to keep the organic compound catecholamine active for prolonged periods of time. This compound is similar to adrenaline is some ways. If you have POTS, remember to be cautious when using over-the-counter commodities to stay safe.

- **Lethargy** – Persons who have been diagnosed with POTS should live their own lives and make sure they are always comfortable with what they do. The point is that you should move at your own pace if you have the syndrome. Just like other triggers, fatigue can lead to more venous pooling. Those suffering from POTS should make the necessary lifestyle changes to avoid worsening the condition. For example, you should avoid the strenuous activities you used to engage in before you developed the syndrome.

- **Balloon Blowing** – When you blow a balloon, you have to force air out of your lungs and most of the air is carbon dioxide. This may increase some of the symptoms experienced by POTS patients including lightheadedness and dizziness.

If you have the symptoms of POTS, you will have difficulty completing your everyday tasks. A proper diagnosis is needed to rule out other conditions, but sometimes the symptoms may be mistaken for low blood pressure. Although we did not talk about low blood pressure as one of the symptoms of POTS, you or the person suffering from the syndrome should consult a doctor for more information. The doctor will perform an accurate diagnosis of the problem and help you or your loved one make the necessary adjustments to alleviate the symptoms.

Research findings regarding the treatment for POTS show that some patients can manage the triggers and symptoms through lifestyle adjustments. Certain medications may be useful, but they are usually recommended if other interventions have failed. If the patient has to use medication, then it is important to work together with a physician. With a detailed guide like this book, those suffering from POTS, including people who have never heard of the syndrome before, can easily manage the condition and find the most suitable solution for their problem.

CHAPTER 3:

Causes and Types of POTS

Causes of POTS

Many breakthroughs in the field of medicine have inspired practitioners to learn more about the causes of different types of illnesses and syndromes. With the help of research, modern-day practitioners can use a wide range of medications for diseases and have established diagnostic procedures to evaluate symptoms. However, it is important to acknowledge that researchers and practitioners are yet to find the causes of certain conditions including Postural Tachycardia Syndrome.

Even after 20 years of extensive medical research on POTS, it is still difficult to understand the syndrome for various reasons. One problem with the syndrome is that it can occur along with other health problems. However, researchers and practitioners in the field of medicine have gathered sufficient evidence showing that patients with the symptoms of POTS have a malfunctioning autonomic nervous system. The main function of this system is to regulate the body's involuntary functions such as heartbeat and blood circulation.

POTS is not considered to be a disease because it is characterized by a variety of disorders with similar symptoms. This is why it may not be easy to tell whether a person is suffering from the disorder, and it is fine to say that we are yet to discover the real cause of POTS. In simple terms, those suffering from POTS experience a variety of symptoms that occur together recurrently. A proper diagnosis can be performed by looking at the various symptoms of the syndrome. Patients may experience random symptoms, which differ from one person to another. Also, the causes and symptoms of POTS may not be the same for every patient due to factors like age.

Additionally, the onset is different in different individuals.

As mentioned earlier in this book, many people who are diagnosed with POTS are aged between 15 and 50 years. The bodily changes and rapid growth experienced by young people during puberty could be responsible for the development of POTS in teenagers. According to the available statistics, about 1 out of every 100 teenagers is diagnosed with POTS. Some women have claimed to have increased symptoms of POTS before menstrual periods.

Many people have also claimed to experience the symptoms of POTS after a surgical procedure, pregnancy, viral infection, or traumatic event. According to research on infections, certain viral infections can damage the vasculature. Once the damage occurs, an auto-immune response is triggered leading to the onset of POTS.

When it comes to POTS in children, the majority of them suffer from a genetic health condition known as joint hypermobility syndrome. Those suffering from the syndrome have an extremely elastic vasculature compared to other children. Their vasculature is too elastic to maintain the appropriate tightness level. For some children, it is said that the syndrome is inherited through genes and it only takes a trigger to activate the symptoms. Unfortunately, some of the people who suffer from POTS claim that they have experienced the symptoms for as long as they can remember.

Health Conditions That May Lead to POTS

Research has shown that certain health conditions may play a role in the development of POTS. However, it is vital to note that these conditions may not be the real cause of the syndrome. You need to know about them to learn more about Postural Tachycardia Syndrome, the possible causes of the syndrome, and treatment methods.

Joint Hypermobility Syndrome or JHS is one of the conditions associated with the development of POTS. Persons afflicted with this physical disorder have abnormally elastic blood vessels and their joints tend to be unusually supple. According to studies, most JHS patients have inherited the syndrome.

Inappropriate Sinus Tachycardia or IST is another health condition associated with the onset of POTS. Studies show that IST can lead to the development of the symptoms experienced by those suffering from hyperadrenergic POTS. People with IST often have an abnormally high heart rate compared to that of POTS patients in a supine position. Their heart rate can accelerate quickly because of stress or physical exertion.

Mast Cell Activation Disorder or MCAD has also been associated with the onset of Post Tachycardia Syndrome, especially if the flushing or allergies are protruding. Studies have revealed that genetic mutation is responsible for the development of this disorder because the mutation causes excessive mast cells to develop. These cells are responsible for protecting you from illnesses and have the capability to health wounds naturally. However, in persons with MCAD, large numbers of mast cells around the patient's blood vessels, skin, gastrointestinal tract, urinary tract, and the respiratory tract are potentially dangerous. For instance, these cells can lead to a faster heartbeat, itching, and flushing.

Persons with Chronic Fatigue Syndrome (CFS) are also likely to be affected by POTS compared to the rest of the population. Research findings show that about 33% of patients diagnosed with CFS are at a higher risk of developing POTS. Patients with CFS usually experience chronic tiredness for a long period of time. Just like POTS, health researchers and practitioners are yet to establish the factors responsible for the development of CFS. However, the most common theory claims that CFS is caused by a viral infection. More research is needed to prove this claim.

Types of POTS

As explained earlier in this chapter, POTS is characterized by a set of disorders with the same or similar clinical manifestations. Although there are many classification systems, this section of the chapter will only focus on clinically relevant groups of disorders that are consistent with evidence from current medical research.

The two major categories of Postural Tachycardia Syndrome are primary and secondary POTS. Primary POTS is idiopathic meaning that it occurs spontaneously and the cause is not known. Simply put, primary POTS is not associated with other disease while secondary POTS is related to another health condition.

Primary POTS

Partial Dysautonomic or PD is the most common name for primary Postural Tachycardia Syndrome. Those suffering from PD usually experience mild symptoms of Peripheral Autonomic Neuropathy or PAN. If you have PAN, your peripheral vasculature, especially your nervous system, is unable to constrict properly in the presence of the earth's gravitation pull. This means that patients with PAN are likely to experience more blood pooling than usual. When this happens, the dependent parts of the body including the legs, lower arms, and mesenteric vasculature are more likely to experience blood pooling.

Myocardial contractility happens when the blood is forcefully moved from some of the patient's blood vessels. The main goal is to increase the patient's heart rate and maintain the body's normal cerebral perfusion pressure. However, myocardial contractility and an increase in the heart rate may be compensatory at the outset. More blood pooling may take place over time and even go beyond the compensatory level. Moreover, persons with this condition tend to use their skeletal muscles most of the time to maintain normal blood pressure.

Researchers have inferred that the origin of the primary type of POTS is immune-mediated. Many of the patients with this form of POTS claim to experience the symptoms immediately after a severe febrile illness. This may happen after a viral illness, immunization, traumatic events, surgical procedures, pregnancy, and sepsis. It is estimated that 5 out of every 6 patients with primary Postural Tachycardia Syndrome are females. However, this is just a rough estimate so additional research is needed to get an accurate figure.

Secondary POTS

The secondary form of POTS is also known as hyperadrenergic POTS. This type of POTS is not as common as primary POTS. Secondary POTS may also refer to a wide range of conditions that lead to peripheral autonomic unresponsiveness accompanied by moderate cardiac tissue innervations.

Studies show that patients with a chronic case of diabetes mellitus are more likely to develop secondary POTS than nondiabetic patients. Other health problems that may lead to secondary POTS include sarcoidosis, alcoholism, amyloidosis, heavy mental intoxication, lupus, and Sjogren's syndrome. People can also develop the secondary form of POTS after undergoing chemotherapy. Joint Hypermobility Syndrome (JHS) is another possible cause of POTS. JHS is a disorder that affects connective tissues and its symptoms include hypermobile and hypertensive joints. Persons with JHS may also have fragile connective tissues.

Research findings show that most of the people who suffer from secondary POTS are adolescents, especially those who experience rapid growth at the age of fourteen. The symptoms of the syndrome worsen within a very short time and usually reach their peak at the age of sixteen. In some cases, these symptoms are extremely devastating making it almost impossible to perform normal tasks. The good news is that these symptoms have been reported to disappear over time. According to studies, about 80% of young adults aged between 19 and 24 years show no symptoms of the syndrome (asymptomatic). There is no clear explanation, but the autonomic imbalance that takes place among members of this group could be one of the reasons.

Research on the symptoms experienced by the rest of the population shows that patients with secondary POTS have symptoms that develop progressively. This means that their symptoms do not occur abruptly. The common symptoms experienced by patients with Hyperadrenergic POTS include tremors, anxiety, and cold extremities when in an upright position. Additionally, reports indicate that about 50% of patients with this form of POTS experience excessive urine output after standing for a short duration. They also complain of headaches and severe migraines.

One of the common characteristics of hyperadrenergic POTS is the development of hypertension and orthostatic tachycardia. Moreover, most patients with this type of POTS have high levels of norepinephrine in their serum (more than 600 ng/ml), especially when they stand up. They are also very responsible to intravenous isoproterenol. Some studies have classified hyperadrenergic POTS as a genetic disorder. According to their findings, a single mutation affects the functions of the transporter protein responsible for clearing norepinephrine from the patient's intrasynaptic cleft. As a result, a spillover of large amounts of norepinephrine serum occurs in response to sympathetic stimuli.

Hypovolemic and Neuropathic POTS

Researchers are still working hard to gather more information about POTS. However, some researchers have a different way of classifying this disorder and some forms of the syndrome are categorized based on their most noticeable characteristics. For example, low blood volume is the major characteristic of hypovolemic POTS while autonomic neuropathy is the key characteristic of neuropathic POTS. Many patients with POTS have two or three characteristics including low blood volume and autonomic neuropathy, which cannot be considered to be distinct circumstances.

CHAPTER 4:

Diagnosing Postural Tachycardia Syndrome

One of the reasons why people misdiagnose POTS is the fact that those suffering from the syndrome may show a wide range of symptoms. These symptoms are similar to the ones exhibited by patients with other health problems including depression, anxiety, and chronic fatigue syndrome. POTS appeared in journals for the first time in 1993, but many health practitioners are still not aware of the syndrome.

Another problem with the symptoms of POTS is that they can change every day. This change causes ambiguities and makes it difficult to carry out an accurate diagnosis of the condition. Patients with

POTS may experience mild, bad or severe symptoms. Doctors may also rule out POTS because they often measure the patient's heart rate and blood pressure while the patient is sitting down. The truth is that the doctor may get normal readings when the patient is sitting down. For this reason, doctors should also gather the necessary data while the patient is standing.

A general practitioner may diagnose the syndrome, but they may ask you to look for a specialist to perform an accurate diagnosis of POTS. You can find a specialist in cardiology or syncope clinics. There are different types of specialists in this field including neurologists, hospital physicians, and heart rhythm specialists. Your doctor or specialist will ask you detailed questioned to gather information about your experiences and symptoms in order to diagnose POTS accurately. The practitioner will also try to find out the possible causes and carry out the necessary physical examinations and investigations.

Criteria for an Accurate Diagnosis of POTS

The following factors must be considered to perform an accurate diagnosis of POTS:

- Blood pressure does not drop when the patient is in an upright position
- Heart rate increases by more than 40 bpm for patients aged between 12 and 19 years
- Heart rate increases by more than 30 bpm after standing for 10 minutes

Note: These factors may not apply if the patient's normal heart rate is low.

Your physician or specialist may use a variety of tests to perform an accurate diagnosis of the disorder and rule out other disorders with the same symptoms as POTS. Here are the most popular diagnostic procedures for POTS:

Active Stand or Poor Man's Tilt

This is a popular diagnostic procedure for POTS. Your doctor will ask you to rest in a supine position and quickly rise to an upright position. This normally happens in two, five or ten-minute intervals. The doctor will then measure your blood pressure and heart rate. The problem with this procedure is that it can trigger some POTS symptoms including fainting depending on the patient's condition. Therefore, a specialist should supervise the procedure.

Tilt Table

Tilt Table is the most popular test for diagnosing POTS. The test is performed in a calm, dimly lit, and temperature controlled environment. The required tools include a footplate and a special table or bed that can tilt upright (60o to 75o). Your physician will ask you to lie down and strap you to the table. The specialist will then record your heart rate and blood pressure. You will stay in a supine position for about

5 to 20 minutes. The physician will then tilt the table to about 60° to 75°. Next, the specialist will look for POTS symptoms and record any changes in your heart rate and blood pressure.

You may be asked to tell the specialist what you are feeling. The information you share will help the doctors perform an accurate interpretation of your blood pressure and heart rate readings. When performing the Tilt Table Test, the best results are usually achieved by doing the test for about forty to forty-five minutes. The doctor will also conclude the test if you faint or experience low blood pressure.

24-Hour BP and Heart Rate Monitoring

When doing this test, the doctor will attach patches and other small devices to your chest. The devices are attached to a light-weight box, which is then attached to your waist using a belt. Your doctor can use one of these devices to monitor your heart rate for 24 hours. Another device will be attached to your arm to measure your blood pressure during that period. You will be required to carry out your everyday activities and avoid any activity that could be responsible for your symptoms. The doctors will check the readings to determine whether your blood pressure drops or your heart rate increases when the symptoms of POTS start to manifest. Usually, your doctor will ask you to keep a diary with information about the time when the symptoms manifested and what you were doing at that time.

Isoproterenol Administration

Isoproterenol is a type of drug that your doctor may administer to determine the type of POTS you are suffering from. The main purpose of using this drug is to test the patient's beta-receptor sensitivity. Generally, this drug tends to increase the symptoms of POTS in patients with the hyperadrenergic form of POTS and beta-receptor sensitivity.

24-Hour Urine Test

As the name suggests, this test involves collecting the patient's urine for a period of 24 hours. Doctors use the urine to test sodium and plasma levels in patients with POTS. Another urine test may be performed to find out whether the patient has increased levels of noradrenaline and epinephrine. This test is useful because it helps the doctor to establish whether Pheochromocytoma (adrenal gland tumor) is the cause of POTS symptoms or not.

Blood Tests

Blood tests will help your doctor rule out other health problems that may be present in your body. These tests can be used to test your glucose levels, kidney function, liver function, thyroid function, and blood count. Hypovolemia or low blood volume may also be checked because it can occur in persons with POTS. The doctor may also check your plasma volume levels and red blood cell mass to find out whether they are normal.

Heart Ultrasound (Echocardiogram)

An ultrasound of the heart is a simple, painless, and harmless test similar to the one performed on expectant women to create an image of the unborn baby. Doctors can use this test on POTS patients to check their heart structure. To perform a heart ultrasound scan, your doctor will apply some jelly on your chest and roll the ultrasound probe on your skin. He or she will move the probe in all directions to produce a 3-dimensional image of your heart on the screen. The doctor will look at the image to determine if your heart is normal.

Microneurography

This is a neurophysiological test performed by scientists and health practitioners to record an individual's postganglionic sympathetic neural traffic from peripheral muscles and the skin. Doctors can perform this test on patients with POTS and symptoms of nerve damage in the legs. Your doctor will place a thin needle into one of your leg nerves to record traffic from your peripheral nerves.

Holter Monitor

In medicine, a Holter monitor is a portable, battery-operated device or an electrocardiography device used by doctors to record a patient's heart activity. The patient is required to wear the device for at least 24 hours during the test. If you have POTS, your doctor can use this device to determine if you have sinus tachycardia. The portable recorder checks for irregular heartbeats and the data recorded during the test allows the doctor to learn more about your heart's activity. This test may also involve placing electrodes at different parts of your chest.

Hand Grip Test

This is one of the simplest, non-invasive tests for measuring the patient's blood pressure. It involves squeezing a handgrip for some time until the patient's hands feel fatigued. If the patient's diastolic pressure is extremely high, they could be having autonomic dysfunction. The Hand Grip Test is suitable for testing the patient's sympathetic function. Some medical practitioners claim that this test is more sensitive than the Tilt Table Test.

Sweat Tests

Abnormal sweating is one of the problems experienced by some patients who have been diagnosed with POTS. This often occurs during the night because many POTS patients have problems with their body's sweat mechanisms. One way to determine if a POTS patient is sweating inappropriately is to carry out a sweat test. There are different options to choose from including the resting sweat output test, thermoregulatory test, and the Quantitative Sudomotor Axon Reflex Test or QSART. Your doctor will choose the appropriate sweat test for you if necessary.

The selected sweat test will help your doctor check some of the possible indicators of POTS. For example, the Quantitative Sudomotor Axon Reflex Test can be used to measure your sweat volume as well as response latency. On the other hand, the thermoregulatory test is suitable if the doctor wants to examine your sweating patterns to identify abnormalities. When using this test, the doctor applies some powder to your skin. Usually, the patient wears a disposable bathing suit as the doctor applies the orange powder.

Once the required amount of powder is applied to your body, your body will be exposed to hot temperatures to induce sweating. When your body starts to sweat, the powder changes from orange to purple helping the doctor identify the sweating parts of your body. The resting sweat output test involves using a battery-operated device to produce an electric current. Doctors perform this test to stimulate the patient's sweat glands.

Stress Test

The stress test allows doctors to find out how the patient's body reacts to exercises. If your doctor decides to carry out this test, you'll be asked to walk on a treadmill. Your physician will keep a record of your heart's electrical activity as you walk on the treadmill and the exercise will continue until you reach the desired heart rate. The exercise ends the moment you become tired. In addition to recording the heart's electrical activity, the doctor may decide to perform a heart ultrasound or echocardiogram during the exercise.

Catecholamine Test

In some cases, doctors may use the Catecholamine test to determine if a POTS patient has chemical abnormalities. The adrenal glands produce hormones known as catecholamines, which are released to the patient's bloodstream when the patient is under emotional or physical stress. The common types of these hormones include dopamine, epinephrine, and norepinephrine. Some of the people diagnosed with POTS have unusual levels of catecholamines, especially the hormone norepinephrine. This hormone is the sympathetic nervous system's primary chemical courier. Doctors can use the 24-hour urine test or perform tests on the patient's blood to measure catecholamine levels.

As you and your doctor look for the appropriate tests to determine if you have POTS, bear in mind that the tests described here should only be used if the doctor thinks you have the symptoms of POTS or autonomic dysfunction. Additionally, those diagnosed with POTS should first consult their doctor if they want to stop medication after undergoing specific tests.

Chapter 5:

Lifestyle Adjustments and Medications for POTS

The first thing that might happen when a person is diagnosed with Postural Tachycardia Syndrome is to feel sad or frustrated. However, if your doctor tells you that you have POTS, there is no need to worry about it because there is a solution. You can easily get yourself out of trouble by making the recommended lifestyle changes. These include a wide range of activities that have proven to be effective in alleviating and curing the symptoms POTS.

Physical activities are among the major factors to consider when it comes to lifestyle adjustments for POTS patients. You will be required to make certain changes until you recover from POTS even if it means avoiding some of the things you have been doing every day. In general, POTS is not a life-threatening condition, but you need to know more about the syndrome so you can manage it, become productive, and restore your happiness.

Lifestyle Adjustments

We have already learned that persons afflicted with POTS experience the symptoms associated with the syndrome in different ways due to different factors. If you have been diagnosed with the condition, it is vital to consult your physician for assistance. Work together with your physician to manage the condition and improve your overall health.

Here are some of the common lifestyle adjustments for managing and curing the syndrome:

Drink More Fluids Regularly

Patients with POTS can alleviate the symptoms of the condition by drinking large amounts of fluids regularly. As mentioned earlier, dehydration can aggravate the symptoms by lowering the patient's blood volume levels. If you are experiencing the symptoms of POTS, you can boost your blood volume levels by drinking 2-3 liters of fluid every day. You should also consider drinking more fluids before you get out of your bed in the morning. This is necessary because the symptoms of POTS may worsen in the morning. Also, remember to take 2 glasses of water if you feel like the symptoms are worsening. This helps to boost low blood pressure and heart rate.

Another important factor to consider when drinking fluids is the type of fluid you want to use. Some drinks are not suitable for POTS patients because they can worsen the symptoms. Caffeinated drinks can worsen the symptoms for certain patients. POTS patients should also avoid alcohol because it can cause hypotension by dilating blood vessels. Additionally, those diagnosed with POTS should do some research to know the possible effects of the dairy products they consume. Some of these products may have a negative impact on the patient's condition. If you realize that some dairy products make you more symptomatic, make sure your meals include other sources of calcium. Remember to consult a doctor and ask them about the fluids you need to drink to manage your condition.

Maintain Good Body Posture

Watch out for the onset of certain signs like lightheadedness, nausea, and dizziness to reduce the risk of fainting. If you experience these symptoms, the first thing you need to do is to rest in a supine position while elevating your legs. If you find it difficult to stay in this position, just stand and try to cross your legs, or rock down or up on your toes. Another way to avoid fainting is to avoid sitting or standing for prolonged periods. If you have been sitting for a while, don't stand abruptly. Stand up slowly to reduce the chances of fainting.

Increase Salt Intake

One of the recommended steps for managing POTS is to increase salt intake. The appropriate amount ranges from 3,000 to 10,000 milligrams of salt per day. If necessary, your doctor will prescribe salt tablets. Extra fluid and salt can be useful for patients who sweat more or feel hot. As you increase your salt intake, remember that high amounts of salt may have negative effects on the body if you have hypertension, heart disease, or kidney disease. The best way to know whether you can consume more salt is to see your doctor for advice.

Eat the Right Foods

The foods and the amount of food you eat may affect your condition in various ways. For instance, your POTS symptoms may worsen if you consume large amounts of food. This is because the body directs blood to your digestive system leaving other areas with insufficient amounts of blood. Instead of having 3 or 4 large meals every day, try to have small, regular meals. POTS patients should also avoid certain types of foods including foods with high amounts of sugar and white flour content. Such foods contain refined carbohydrates, which are known to aggravate the symptoms of POTS in some people. The best foods for persons with POTS include unprocessed foods like beans, whole grains, vegetables, and fruits.

Regulate Temperatures

Heat is not good for POTS patients because it can worsen the symptoms. If the environment around you is humid, spray your neck and face with some water. You can also avoid hot temperatures by staying in air-conditioned buildings. Another effective way of regulating your body temperature is to have cloth layers. You can easily remove the top layers to inhibit overheating.

Wear Compression Clothing

One way to reduce the symptoms of POTS is to increase the flow of blood in your legs. Try out some compression clothing like tights to keep the blood flowing. The selected clothing should reach your waist. Also, the pressure at the ankles should be 30 mm HG or more to achieve the best results.

Elevate Your Head during Sleep

Some POTS patients cannot sleep well at night due to the effects of POTS symptoms. Depression and anxiety are some of the factors responsible for poor sleep among these patients. If you are having sleep problems because of the symptoms of POTS, you should avoid sleeping flat. Try to stack several pillows or soft objects and use them to elevate your head while sleeping. This will allow blood to reach the lower parts of your body during the night or whenever you feel like sleeping.

Match Physical Activities with Your Capabilities

As discussed earlier in this book, strenuous physical activities can aggravate the symptoms associated with POTS. Physical exertion makes it more difficult to recover and may extend your recovery time. For this reason, people with the syndrome should only engage in moderate exercises. This may help to relieve the symptoms and cure the condition. The main objective of engaging in such exercises is to strengthen the patient's core muscles and legs. Strong core muscles help to pump blood from various parts of the body to your heart.

In case you have not been taking part in any form of physical activity and you have POTS, you should first try some recumbent exercises. These exercises are done while lying or sitting down. Keep exercising and increase the duration gradually provided that your body can handle the pressure. Continue until you can do the exercises in an upright position. It usually takes about 2 to 3 months of recumbent exercises to reach a point where you can exercise in this position.

If the physical exercises you have been performing have produced good results, try some aerobic exercises between 20 and 30 minutes long. Do these exercises 2 or 3 times every week and include some calisthenics and resistance training if possible. The most common forms of exercises for people with POTS symptoms include walking, rowing, jogging, swimming, and resistance training on lower-limb muscles. These exercises play a crucial role in strengthening your calf muscles making it easier for blood to flow back to your heart. They also keep POTS patients physically fit and healthy.

Manage Personal Hygiene

If you have been diagnosed with POTS, avoid taking hot and long baths to reduce the risk of dilating your blood vessels or aggravating the symptoms. When showering, try to always finish with cold water to alleviate POTS symptoms. In addition, consider sitting on something like a stool while in the shower because you may worsen the symptoms if you stand for a long time. Don't forget to take some fluids after and before the shower. If the weather is dry, feel free to use shampoo sprays and wet wipes.

Plan in Advance

Many POTS patients say that their symptoms tend to worsen in the morning and that is why it is important to plan your day in advance. In other words, you should plan for tomorrow today. As you plan in advance, remember to include your resting time on your list of activities. You don't want to complete your tasks hurriedly if you have POTS.

Adopt Good Work and Reading Habits

If you have some work to do and books to read, you need to avoid brain fog. You can avoid it by keeping your feet elevated when reading or working. Do not procrastinate if you don't want to experience more stress. The people around you in your place of work and school need to know about the possible triggers. The best way to let them know about the triggers is to make a list and help them understand how these factors aggravate the symptoms of POTS. This will also keep you away from trouble when you are around other people.

Use a Mobility Scooter or Wheelchair

While some POTS patients are strong enough to take part in different types of exercises, some patients are not able to engage in such activities for one reason or the other. However, this does not mean that all bed-ridden patients cannot do their everyday activities. Some of them can do their daily activities with the help of a mobility scooter or wheelchair. These machines are helpful if the patient is too sick to move, or has a sudden outburst of POTS symptoms. Also, mobility scooters and wheelchairs allow you to rest and protect you from the negative effects of continuous physical exertion.

Keep Your Tools in One Place

Patients with POTS have to use a variety of tools to manage the symptoms of their condition. This means that you can easily feel exhausted in an attempt to gather everything you need once you are diagnosed with the disorder. The last thing you want to do if you have POTS is to waste the energy to need to perform the most important tasks. You may also have trouble picking up the tools you need to use throughout the day, especially if they are not in one place. To avoid this, place the items you need in a purse or knapsack before you leave the house. You should avoid wasting your energy just because you are unable to find things like your POTS medicine, salt, and water bottle.

List Your Medication and Create Reminders

Lastly, you should list all current POTS medicines along with the appropriate dosages. Remember to create a timetable and reminders to help you take your medicine at the right time. Sometimes the symptoms may become severe, so it is advisable to include your address and contact number. Other useful details include drug and food allergies.

Medications for POTS

Some patients need some form of medication to reduce the negative effects of POTS symptoms. Medical practitioners will tell you that there is no single medicinal treatment for POTS and it is not easy to treat the condition successfully. This is probably because persons with POTS experience the symptoms differently meaning that each medication plan is unique to each patient. In addition, the effects of POTS medication are different for each patient. For example, the medication might aggravate the symptoms, help the patient recover, or have no significant effects on the patient's condition. The main purpose of prescription medicine is not to cure POTS, but to control the symptoms and promote the patient's overall wellbeing.

The recommended treatment regimen is to start with small doses because some POTS patients are extremely sensitive to drugs. Those taking POTS medication should keep an eye on the possible side effects. Some patients try many drugs hoping to get the right treatment, but this can lead to frustrations. The truth is, no single medication has been licensed as an effective treatment for POTS.

Your doctor may decide to prescribe "off-license/label" medicines including the following:

Drugs to Regulate Heart Rate

These drugs include beta blockers (beta-adrenergic blocking agents), ivabradine, alpha agonist, and midodrine. Here is a summary of the drugs:

- **Beta Blockers** – A doctor may prescribe beta blockers to a POTS patient to restore normal blood pressure if it is too high. These drugs may help people with high levels of norepinephrine. Some of these drugs affect the patient's heart while others affect the heart and blood vessels. The problem with beta blockers is that they can affect plasma renin activity (PRA). Low PRA levels are common in hypovolemic orthostatic intolerant individuals. The most popular beta blockers for POTS patients include Metoprolol, Bisoprolol, Labetalol, and Propranolol. Labetalol is said to induce alpha and beta blockade.

- **Ivabradine** – This sinus node blocker can reduce heart rate without dilating the patient's blood vessels, sexual disturbances, or adverse entropic effects.

- **Midodrine** – Midodrine is a popular drug for treating patients with health problems like POTS, hypotension, and fainting. It can stimulate adrenergic receptors and increase blood pressure by narrowing blood vessels. Patients should take it in 2 to 4-hour intervals. The first drug should be taken 1 hour before you leave the bed, while the last drug should be taken 4 hours before going to bed. Midodrine may cause hypertension when the patient is in a supine position. The effects do not last for a long time, so it is important to take it 4 hours before sleeping to prevent hypertension.

- **Alpha Agonist** – This natural substance acts on cellular alpha-adrenoceptors.

- **Serotonin–Noradrenalin Reuptake Inhibitor (SNRI) and Selective Serotonin Reuptake Inhibitor (SSRI)** – These drugs may be used to treat autonomic disorders and that is why they are suitable for POTs patients. They can be used to manage depression and anxiety. The most popular SSRI medications include Sertraline, Escitalopram, and Paroxetine, while the most common SNRI mediations include Venlafaxine, Duloxetine, and Atomoxetine. These drugs can interact and cause complications, so you should consult your doctor. SSRI and SNRI medications may help persons with POTS because these people are thought to have problems with serotonin production and regulation. The human body can produce serotonin, which plays an important role in regulating the heart and blood pressure. Some people claim that SSRI medications improve irritable bowel syndrome symptoms while SNRI medications decrease the reuptake of serotonin and noradrenaline. However, there are significant negative effects including dry mouth, joint pain, nausea, muscle pain, numbness (feet and hands), poor vision, sexual dysfunction, and tinnitus.

Medications to Boost Blood Volume

- **Erythropoietin** – This drug can increase red blood cell (RBC) mass, regulate blood pressure, and make blood vessels narrow. It is good for POTS patients with low RBC levels. Erythropoietin is not common because many patients cannot afford it and it is administered through an injection.

- **Fludrocortisone** – This synthetic steroid can boost plasma levels and retain water and salt. Its effects are different from the effects of prednisolone and other steroids, which is why some patients are cautious. Also, fludrocortisone depletes potassium and magnesium, so it is important to add supplements.

- **Desmopressin (DDVAP)** – DDVAP can reduce the risk of hypotension in the morning and raise blood pressure. The hormone Vasopressin is a synthetic version of DDVAP used to promote fluid retention and reduce urine production in order to increase heart rate.

- **Cerefolin** – Autonomic dysfunction patients can use this vitamin supplement to reduce fatigue and become more alert.

CHAPTER 6:

POTS Prognosis

The long-term outlook or prognosis for persons with POTS is generally good despite the absence of adequate data. Doctors and other health practitioners need to find a uniform outcome in all patients regardless of the diverse manifestations and effects of the syndrome. The current prognosis of the condition is based on observations about what happened to people who have recovered from POTS.

According to the observations, more than 50% of patients diagnosed with the condition showed significant signs of recovery within a period of two to five years. Prognosis is generally better for adolescents, which means young people are likely to recover faster than the rest of the population. Here, the term "recovery" means the lack of orthostatic symptoms as well as being able to perform everyday physical activities with minimal restraint.

The good news is, most of the patients who suffer from POTS (about 90%) recover from the syndrome when using treatment methods that involve physical therapies and pharmacotherapy. However, secondary hyperadrenergic POTS patients may need more therapy to achieve good results. This is necessary because the underlying health problems need to be treated to alleviate the symptoms.

With the increasing number of people who have been diagnosed with POTS, specialists are working hard to learn more about the syndrome. Hopefully, the prognosis for POTS will improve over time.

Conclusion

In this book, you have learned everything you need to know about Postural Tachycardia Syndrome. You will benefit from the information presented here if you have POTS, or use it to help other people who have been affected by the syndrome. I would like to express my gratitude for purchasing and reading this book. Hopefully, you have obtained the information you needed to understand what POTS is and learned how to manage the syndrome and help other POTS patients. The book has covered the basics of POTS and it is my wish that it will guide you and other readers who want to learn more about the syndrome and the recommended solutions to alleviate the symptoms.

Medical history shows that humans were aware of POTS even before the year 1993 when medical practitioners claimed to have conducted research on the syndrome. The truth about POTS is that it can affect all people regardless of their age, race, and gender. However, some studies show that women are 5 times more likely to develop POTS than men. Also, the syndrome can develop in healthy individuals. I believe that this book has helped you understand why you or your loved one can or has experienced the symptoms of POTS.

Hopefully, you have learned about the most common symptoms exhibited by those suffering from POTS. You can use this knowledge to help others identify the symptoms. If you notice any of the symptoms described in this book, make sure you see a doctor and advise others with the symptoms to do the same. Whether you or someone else is the patient, it is important to know the symptoms of the syndrome and prevent triggers that are known to worsen the condition. POTS patients may have different symptoms and the people around you will appreciate it if you can spot the symptoms of the condition and provide some basic knowledge about the condition.

This book will also act as a guide to help you make the necessary life adjustments and take the appropriate steps if you are suffering from POTS. It is a good resource or reference book for the various tests, medications, and treatments for the syndrome. Make the most of the information presented here so you could live a normal life.

Although POTS is not a life-threatening health problem, a misdiagnosis can have devastating effects on your health and life. It can lead to serious complications and this is what we are trying to avoid. If you have the condition, make sure you get in touch and work with your physician through the entire treatment process.

Finally, I would like to thank you once more for purchasing and reading this book. I hope you have found the information you needed to help yourself and other people who might be suffering from POTS.